Living with Colon Cancer

A Personal Journey of Triumph and Hope

Gina J. Hughes

All rights reserved. No part of this publication may be reproduced, distributed, or transmitted in any form or by any means, including photocopying, recording, or other electronic or mechanical methods without the publisher's prior written permission, except in the case of brief quotation embodied in critical reviews permitted by copyright law.

Table Of Content

Introduction

When I was diagnosed with colon cancer, my world was turned upside down. At the age of 42, I was suddenly faced with a life-threatening illness that would require aggressive treatment and a complete upheaval of my daily routine. The road ahead seemed daunting, filled with uncertainty and fear.

But as I began my journey through cancer treatment, I discovered something that surprised me: a deep well of inner strength that I never knew I had. Through the pain, the discomfort, and the emotional turmoil, I found myself drawing on reserves of courage and resilience that I never knew existed.

As I navigated the ups and downs of my cancer journey, I felt compelled to share my story with others. I wanted to provide hope and encouragement to those who were facing similar challenges, and to offer practical advice on how to cope with the physical and emotional toll of cancer treatment.

In this book, "Living with Colon Cancer: A Personal Journey of Triumph and Hope," I share my story of facing cancer head-on and emerging on the other side with a renewed appreciation for life. I talk about the diagnosis, the treatment, the recovery, and the spiritual and emotional growth that came from my experience.

Whether you are currently facing cancer yourself, or are supporting a loved one who is, I hope that my story will offer you comfort, inspiration, and practical guidance. I believe that even in the darkest of times, there is hope, and that by sharing our stories, we can find strength and support in one another.

In the pages of this book, you'll find a candid account of what it's really like to live with colon cancer. I don't sugarcoat the reality of the disease, and I share the difficult moments as well as the triumphs. But ultimately, this is a story of hope and resilience, of finding light in the darkness, and of discovering a newfound appreciation for the gift of life.

Along the way, I offer practical advice on how to cope with the physical and emotional challenges of cancer treatment. From managing side effects of chemotherapy and surgery to finding emotional support and spiritual comfort, I share what worked for me and what I learned from my experience.

I also discuss the role of faith in my journey and how I found meaning in suffering. Whether or not you are a religious person, I hope that my reflections on spirituality and the search for purpose will resonate with you and offer you insight into your own life journey.

Finally, I talk about life after cancer and how I've learned to embrace a new sense of purpose and meaning. I share my thoughts on coping with the fear of recurrence, the importance of follow-up care, and the joys of rediscovering everyday pleasures after a life-altering experience.

It is my hope that by sharing my story, I can offer hope and encouragement to others who are facing cancer, and that I can help to raise awareness about this disease and the importance of early detection and treatment. Thank you for joining me on this journey, and I hope that my story will inspire you to find strength, hope, and meaning in your own life, no matter what challenges you may face.

Chapter 1: Diagnosis

The Shock of Hearing "You Have Cancer"

I'll never forget the day I received my diagnosis. It was a routine check-up with my primary care physician, and I had no reason to suspect that anything was wrong. But after a series of tests, my doctor sat me down and delivered the news: I had colon cancer.

At first, I was in shock. It felt like the ground had been pulled out from under me, and I could hardly comprehend what I was hearing. Cancer was something that happened to other people, not to me. How could this be happening?

As I left the doctor's office, I felt numb and disoriented. The world around me seemed to be moving in slow motion, and I could hardly process what was happening. I knew that I needed to tell my loved ones, but the thought of breaking the news to them was almost too much to bear.

The Diagnostic Process

After the initial shock wore off, I was faced with a whirlwind of doctor's appointments and tests. I quickly learned that diagnosing cancer is a complex and often lengthy process, and that there were many steps to take before we would know the full extent of my illness.

First came the consultations with specialists: a gastroenterologist, an oncologist, and a surgeon. Each one explained what their role would be in my treatment and what I could expect in the weeks and months ahead. I felt overwhelmed by the amount of information I was receiving, and it was difficult to keep everything straight.

Next came the tests. There were blood tests, stool tests, and imaging tests like CT scans and MRIs. Each one seemed to reveal something new, and the results were often conflicting or inconclusive. It was hard to know what to make of all the data, and I found myself constantly second-guessing whether I was making the right decisions.

Coping with Fear and Uncertainty

Throughout the diagnostic process, I was plagued by fear and uncertainty. Would the cancer be contained to my colon, or had it spread to other parts of my body? How would I cope with the physical and emotional toll of treatment? What would happen to my family and my job?

It was hard to find answers to these questions, and I often felt like I was in a fog of uncertainty. But as I began to tell my loved ones about my diagnosis, I discovered a surprising source of comfort: the support and encouragement of those around me.

My family and friends rallied around me, offering words of comfort and practical help. They helped me make sense of the medical jargon and navigate the healthcare system. They were there to listen when I needed to vent, and to offer a shoulder to cry on when the emotions became overwhelming.

As I look back on that time now, I realize that the diagnostic process was just the beginning of my cancer journey. But it was also a time of profound growth and transformation. In the face of fear and uncertainty, I discovered a well of inner strength and resilience that I never knew existed. And I learned that, with the support of loved ones, there was nothing I couldn't face.

I also discovered the power of advocacy and self-education. As I navigated the healthcare system and worked with my medical team, I realized that I needed to be an active participant in my own care. I read books, researched online, and talked to others who had been through similar experiences. I asked questions, challenged assumptions, and sought out second opinions when necessary.

Through it all, I began to see myself not just as a cancer patient, but as a survivor. I knew that the road ahead would be long and difficult, but I also felt a sense of hope and determination. I was determined to fight this disease with everything I had, and to come out the other side stronger and more resilient than ever before.

In the coming chapters of this book, I'll share more about my journey with colon cancer: the ups and downs of treatment, the challenges of recovery, and the joys of life after cancer. But for now, I hope that my story will offer comfort and support to anyone who is going through a similar experience.

If you've recently received a cancer diagnosis, I want you to know that you are not alone. You have a team of medical professionals, family, friends, and even strangers who are there to support you through this difficult time. And I hope that this book will offer you insight, inspiration, and encouragement as you navigate your own cancer journey.

Together, we can face this disease with courage, compassion, and hope.

Chapter 2

Treatment Options

Understanding Your Treatment Options
After my diagnosis, one of the first questions on my mind was: how do we treat this thing? I had a vague idea of what cancer treatment entailed, but I had no real understanding of the different options that were available to me.

As I began to research and ask questions, I discovered that there were three main types of treatment for colon cancer: surgery, chemotherapy, and radiation therapy. Each option had its own benefits and drawbacks, and each required careful consideration and consultation with my medical team.

Surgery: The Gold Standard for Colon Cancer Treatment

For most patients with colon cancer, surgery is the first line of treatment. The goal of surgery is to remove the cancerous tumor and any surrounding tissue that may be affected. Depending on the location and size of the tumor, this may involve removing a portion of the colon or the entire colon.

As I considered surgery, I had many questions: What would the procedure involve? How long would the recovery take? What would the long-term effects be? My surgeon patiently answered all of my questions, and helped me to understand what to expect before, during, and after the surgery.

Chemotherapy: What It Is and How It Works

Chemotherapy is a treatment that uses drugs to kill cancer cells. These drugs are usually administered intravenously, and can be given in a variety of schedules and doses depending on the patient's needs.

As I learned more about chemotherapy, I was apprehensive about the potential side effects. Would I lose my hair? Would I be constantly nauseous and fatigued? My oncologist reassured me that while there were certainly side effects to be aware of, many patients were able to manage them with medication and lifestyle changes.

Radiation Therapy: When and How It's Used

Radiation therapy uses high-energy rays or particles to kill cancer cells. It's often used in conjunction with surgery or chemotherapy to target cancer cells that may have spread beyond the primary tumor.

While radiation therapy sounded intimidating at first, my radiation oncologist helped me to understand the process and the potential benefits. We discussed the potential side effects, and worked together to create a treatment plan that would be best suited to my needs.

Making Treatment Decisions

As I weighed my options for treatment, I found myself considering not just the medical factors, but also my personal preferences and priorities. Did I want to prioritize quality of life, or take a more aggressive approach to treatment? Was I willing to tolerate certain side effects in exchange for a better chance of long-term survival?

Ultimately, I decided to undergo surgery followed by chemotherapy. While the treatment was certainly challenging, I felt a sense of empowerment in knowing that I was taking an active role in my own care.

The Agony Of Chemotherapy

Chemotherapy was easily one of the most difficult experiences of my life. It felt like a never-ending cycle of sickness, fatigue, and pain.

The first time I went in for treatment, I was terrified. I didn't know what to expect, but I knew it wouldn't be easy. The nurse hooked me up to an IV and began administering the drugs. At first, I didn't feel anything. But within a few minutes, I started to feel a strange sensation in my stomach.

Nausea hit me like a ton of bricks. I felt like I was going to throw up, but nothing came out. The nurse gave me some medication to help with the nausea, but it didn't do much. I spent the next few hours feeling miserable, trying to keep my mind off the pain and discomfort.

As the days went on, the side effects of chemotherapy became more and more pronounced. I lost my appetite, and everything I ate tasted bland and unappetizing. I was constantly tired, even though I had trouble sleeping at night. My skin became dry and itchy, and I developed a rash on my arms and legs.

But perhaps the worst part of chemotherapy was losing my hair. I knew it was a possibility, but I didn't realize how much it would affect me emotionally. Seeing myself in the mirror without hair made me feel like a completely different person. I didn't recognize myself, and I felt like I was losing a part of my identity.

Despite all of these challenges, I knew that chemotherapy was my best chance at beating colon cancer. I tried to focus on the positive aspects of treatment, like the fact that the drugs were working to kill cancer cells in my body. I also leaned heavily on my support system, including my family and friends, who helped me get through the toughest days.

Looking back on my experience with chemotherapy, I can honestly say that it was one of the hardest things I've ever gone through. But it was also a period of tremendous growth and strength. I learned that I was capable of so much more than I ever thought possible, and that I had the resilience and determination to fight this disease with everything I had.

The Decision to Have Surgery

When I was first diagnosed with colon cancer, I felt overwhelmed with decisions. But one of the biggest decisions I had to make was whether or not to have surgery.

My doctor had explained that surgery was the most effective way to remove the cancer from my colon. But the thought of going under the knife terrified me. I knew that surgery carried risks, and I didn't want to put myself through such a traumatic experience unless it was absolutely necessary.

I spent weeks researching my options and weighing the pros and cons. On one hand, surgery offered the best chance of curing my cancer and preventing it from spreading to other parts of my body. On the other hand, it would mean a long recovery period and a significant amount of pain and discomfort.

Finally, after much deliberation, I decided to go ahead with the surgery. I knew that it was the best way to ensure that I could live a long and healthy life, and that the potential benefits outweighed the risks.

The day of the surgery was nerve-wracking. I had to go through several rounds of tests and scans to make sure that I was healthy enough for the procedure. When I was finally wheeled into the operating room, I was shaking with fear.

But the team of doctors and nurses was incredibly supportive and comforting. They talked me through every step of the procedure and made sure that I was as comfortable as possible.

When I woke up from the surgery, I was in a lot of pain. But I also felt a sense of relief that the cancer had been removed from my body. Over the next few days, I slowly regained my strength and began the long process of recovery.

Looking back on my decision to have surgery, I know that it was the right choice for me. It wasn't an easy decision, but it was one that I had to make in order to beat colon cancer and live a healthy life.

Coping with Side Effects

Of course, no cancer treatment is without its side effects. During chemotherapy, I experienced fatigue, nausea, and hair loss. I also had to deal with the emotional toll of treatment, which included anxiety and depression.

But through it all, I learned the importance of self-care and support. I took time to rest when I needed to, and made sure to eat a healthy diet and exercise as much as I was able. I also leaned on my loved ones for emotional support, and sought out a therapist to help me cope with the anxiety and depression.

If you're facing a colon cancer diagnosis and treatment, it's important to know that you're not alone. There are many resources available to help you navigate this difficult time, from medical professionals to support groups to online forums.

Navigating the Healthcare System

Navigating the healthcare system can be a daunting task, especially when you're dealing with a serious illness like colon cancer. There are so many doctors, appointments, and treatments to keep track of, and it can be overwhelming to try to stay on top of everything.

In my experience, the key to navigating the healthcare system is to be proactive and informed. I made sure to ask lots of questions and take notes during my appointments, so that I could keep track of all the important details. I also did a lot of research on my own, using online resources and support groups to learn more about my diagnosis and treatment options.

Another important aspect of navigating the healthcare system is finding a doctor that you trust and feel comfortable with. I was fortunate to have an excellent oncologist who was always available to answer my questions and provide guidance. I also made sure to communicate my needs and concerns clearly, so that my doctor could tailor my treatment plan to my specific needs.

It's also important to be organized and keep all of your medical records and paperwork in one place. I created a binder with all of my test results, treatment plans, and medication information, so that I could easily access everything I needed. I also made sure to keep track of my appointments and medications, so that I never missed an important deadline or prescription refill.

Despite the challenges of navigating the healthcare system, I found that it was possible to find my way through the maze with patience and persistence. By staying informed, proactive, and organized, I was able to receive the best possible care and stay on top of my treatment plan.

Chapter 3

<u>*Recovery*</u>

Recovering from colon cancer is a long and often challenging process, both physically and emotionally. In this chapter, I'll share my experience with recovery and offer some tips for managing the ups and downs of life after cancer.

The Physical Recovery

The physical recovery from colon cancer can be difficult, especially if you've undergone surgery or chemotherapy. I found that it was important to listen to my body and take things slow, allowing myself plenty of time to rest and heal.

One of the biggest challenges during my recovery was dealing with the side effects of chemotherapy. I experienced fatigue, nausea, and a loss of appetite, which made it difficult to eat or engage in normal activities. I found that it was helpful to focus on small goals, such as taking a short walk or trying a new food, rather than trying to push myself too hard.

If you've undergone surgery, you may also need to make some adjustments to your daily routine. For example, you may need to avoid lifting heavy objects or engaging in strenuous exercise for several weeks or even months. It can be frustrating to feel limited in this way, but it's important to remember that your body needs time to heal.

The Emotional Recovery

Recovering from colon cancer can also be an emotional journey. After undergoing such a serious illness, it's normal to feel a range of emotions, from fear and anxiety to gratitude and relief.

One of the biggest emotional challenges for me was dealing with the fear of recurrence. Even though I was cancer-free, I found myself constantly worrying about the cancer coming back. It was helpful to talk to other survivors and healthcare professionals about my fears, and to develop a plan for monitoring my health going forward.

Another important aspect of emotional recovery is rebuilding your sense of identity and purpose after cancer. It can be difficult to find your footing after such a traumatic experience, but I found that focusing on my passions and hobbies helped me to regain a sense of normalcy and purpose.

Tips for Recovery

Here are a few tips that helped me during my recovery from colon cancer:

- Be patient and give yourself plenty of time to heal.
- Reach out to other survivors and healthcare professionals for support.
- Stay active and engage in activities that you enjoy.
- Focus on small goals and celebrate your progress.
- Develop a plan for monitoring your health and preventing recurrence.

Recovering from colon cancer is a journey, but with patience, support, and determination, it is possible to regain your health and move forward with your life.

Learning to Ask for Help

As a cancer survivor, I learned that it's important to ask for help when you need it. During recovery, you may find that you need assistance with everyday tasks such as cooking, cleaning, and running errands. It's okay to ask for help from family members, friends, or community organizations.

At first, I struggled with the idea of asking for help. I didn't want to burden anyone or feel like I was being a bother. But as I went through treatment and recovery, I realized that asking for help was a sign of strength, not weakness. It allowed me to focus on my healing and gave others the opportunity to show their love and support.

If you're struggling with asking for help, try to be specific about what you need. Maybe you need someone to drive you to appointments or help with grocery shopping. Maybe you just need someone to talk to when you're feeling down. Whatever it is, don't be afraid to ask. People are often more than happy to help in any way they can.

It's also important to remember that asking for help doesn't mean you're giving up control. You're still in charge of your recovery, and asking for help can actually give you more control by allowing you to focus on your healing and well-being.

In addition to asking for help from loved ones, there are also community resources available for cancer survivors. These might include support groups, counseling services, or organizations that provide financial assistance or transportation.

Remember, you don't have to go through recovery alone. Asking for help is a sign of strength and can help you on your journey towards healing and wellness.

The Importance of Emotional Support

Emotional support is critical during recovery from colon cancer. As a survivor, I found that the emotional toll of cancer was just as challenging as the physical aspects. That's why it's important to seek out emotional support from loved ones, support groups, or mental health professionals.

One of the biggest challenges I faced during recovery was dealing with the emotional aftermath of cancer. I experienced anxiety, depression, and feelings of isolation. It was difficult to talk about my emotions with others, but I knew that it was important to seek out support.

My family and friends were incredibly supportive throughout my recovery journey. They listened to me when I needed to talk, provided encouragement and positive affirmations, and helped me to stay positive. Their emotional support was invaluable in helping me to cope with the challenges of recovery.

In addition to the support of loved ones, I found that joining a support group for cancer survivors was also helpful. It was comforting to talk to others who had been through similar experiences, and it provided a sense of community and connection.

Mental health professionals such as therapists or counselors can also be an important source of emotional support during recovery. They can help you to work through the emotions and challenges that come with cancer, and provide coping strategies and tools to help you manage stress and anxiety.

Remember, it's okay to ask for emotional support when you need it. Recovery from colon cancer can be a rollercoaster of emotions, but with the right support, you can navigate the ups and downs and emerge stronger and more resilient than ever.

Chapter 4

Spiritual and Emotional Growth

Spiritual and emotional growth is an essential component of recovery from colon cancer. Many cancer survivors find that the experience of cancer leads to a deeper understanding of themselves, their relationships, and their place in the world. In this chapter, we will explore how spiritual and emotional growth can help cancer survivors find meaning and purpose in their lives after cancer.

The Role of Spirituality in Recovery

Spirituality can be defined as a belief in a higher power or purpose, and it can play an important role in recovery from cancer. Many cancer survivors find that their faith or spirituality helps them to cope with the challenges of cancer and find meaning in their experiences.

Finding Meaning in Suffering

Suffering is a part of the human experience, and for many cancer survivors, it's an all-too-familiar aspect of the journey. However, despite the challenges of cancer, it's possible to find meaning and purpose in the experience.

For me, finding meaning in my cancer journey was a gradual process. At first, I felt overwhelmed by the physical and emotional toll of the disease. But over time, I began to reflect on what the experience was teaching me about myself and about life.

I realized that cancer had given me a new appreciation for the fragility and preciousness of life. It had taught me to slow down and appreciate the small moments of beauty and joy that make life worth living. It had also helped me to recognize the strength and resilience within myself, and to develop a deeper sense of compassion and empathy for others who were going through their own struggles.

In addition to finding meaning in my own experience, I also found purpose in using my journey to help others. I became involved in cancer support groups and advocacy organizations, using my own experience to support and encourage others who were going through similar struggles.

Ultimately, finding meaning in suffering is a deeply personal and individual process. It may involve exploring one's own beliefs and values, connecting with others who share similar experiences, or simply finding small moments of joy and beauty in the midst of difficulty. But no matter how we find meaning, it's a powerful way to transform suffering into something meaningful and purposeful.

Grappling with Existential Questions

Cancer has a way of forcing us to grapple with some of life's big questions. For many cancer survivors, the experience raises existential questions about the meaning and purpose of life.

I remember the moment when I was diagnosed with cancer. In that instant, everything changed. Suddenly, all of the plans and goals I had for my life were put on hold, and I was faced with the possibility that my time on earth might be limited.

In the days and weeks that followed, I found myself grappling with some deep questions about the meaning and purpose of life. What was the point of all the striving and planning if life could be taken away in an instant? What was the purpose of my own suffering, and how could I make sense of the randomness and unpredictability of life?

As I journeyed through cancer treatment and recovery, I continued to explore these questions. I read books on philosophy and spirituality, seeking guidance and inspiration from those who had wrestled with these questions before me. I talked with others who had experienced cancer, and found comfort and support in their stories of resilience and hope.

Gradually, I began to find my own answers to these questions. I came to realize that the meaning and purpose of life is something that we create for ourselves, through our relationships, our work, and our contributions to the world. I discovered that even in the midst of suffering and uncertainty, there is always the possibility of finding joy and meaning in the present moment.

Today, as a cancer survivor, I continue to grapple with these big questions. But I do so with a greater sense of clarity and purpose, and with a deeper appreciation for the preciousness of life.

The Role of Faith in My Journey

Faith has played a significant role in my cancer journey. As a person of faith, I turned to my beliefs for comfort and strength during some of the most difficult moments of my journey.

In the early days after my diagnosis, I felt overwhelmed and frightened. I struggled to make sense of what was happening to me and to find a sense of peace amid the uncertainty. It was then that I turned to prayer and meditation, seeking a connection with a higher power and a sense of guidance and comfort.

As I underwent treatment and faced the physical and emotional toll of cancer, my faith continued to sustain me. I drew strength from the stories of other people of faith who had faced similar struggles, and I found comfort in the belief that there was a purpose and a plan for my life, even in the midst of suffering.

At times, my faith was tested. There were moments when I felt angry and resentful, questioning why a loving God would allow such suffering to exist in the world. But even in those moments, I continued to cling to my beliefs, recognizing that faith was not about having all the answers, but about finding a sense of peace and hope in the midst of uncertainty.

I have also found that my faith has played a role in shaping my perspective on life after cancer. It has helped me to appreciate the small joys of life and to recognize the importance of living each day to the fullest.

In many ways, my cancer journey has been a spiritual journey as well. It has forced me to confront some of life's big questions and to grapple with the mystery and complexity of the human experience. And while I don't have all the answers, I have found comfort and solace in the belief that there is a higher power at work in the world, guiding us on our journey and giving us the strength and courage to face whatever challenges lie ahead.

For anyone facing a cancer diagnosis, I would encourage them to explore the role of faith in their own journey. Whether through prayer, meditation, or connection with a spiritual community, faith can provide a source of comfort and strength in even the darkest of times. And while it may not provide all the answers, it can help us to find meaning and purpose in the midst of suffering and uncertainty.

Chapter 5

<u>Life After Cancer</u>

Surviving cancer is a major milestone, but it is also just the beginning of a new journey. Life after cancer can be filled with uncertainty, fear, and a range of emotions. For me, it was a time of both joy and apprehension as I learned to navigate the world as a cancer survivor.

Coping with the Fear of Recurrence

One of the biggest challenges that many cancer survivors face is the fear of recurrence. Even after completing treatment and being declared cancer-free, the possibility of the cancer returning can be a source of constant worry and anxiety.

For me, this fear was always lurking in the back of my mind. Every little ache or pain felt like a potential sign of something more serious, and I found myself constantly checking for lumps or abnormalities. The fear was so overwhelming at times that it made it difficult to enjoy life or to plan for the future.

But over time, I learned to manage my anxiety and to cope with the fear of recurrence. One of the things that helped me was staying informed about my cancer and its potential for recurrence. I talked to my doctors about my risk factors and what I could do to reduce my chances of the cancer returning. I also stayed up-to-date on the latest research and treatment options so that I could feel empowered and informed.

Another thing that helped me was practicing mindfulness and staying in the present moment. Rather than constantly worrying about the future, I learned to appreciate the small joys of life and to focus on what was happening in the here and now. Whether it was spending time with loved ones, pursuing a hobby, or simply enjoying a beautiful day, I found that staying present helped me to manage my anxiety and to find a sense of peace.

Of course, there were still times when the fear of recurrence was overwhelming. During those times, I leaned on my support network of family, friends, and fellow survivors. Talking to others who had been through a similar experience helped me to feel less alone and more understood. And when all else failed, I allowed myself to feel my emotions and to grieve for what I had lost.

Today, I still live with the fear of recurrence, but it no longer controls me. I have learned to manage my anxiety and to find ways to cope with the uncertainty that comes with life after cancer. And while the road ahead may be uncertain, I am grateful for each new day and for the opportunity to live a full and meaningful life.

The Importance of Follow-Up Care

After completing cancer treatment, it can be tempting to put the experience behind you and move on with your life. But the truth is, follow-up care is just as important as the initial treatment in ensuring your long-term health and well-being.

For me, follow-up care included regular check-ups with my oncologist, as well as imaging tests and blood work to monitor for any signs of recurrence. While these appointments could be nerve-wracking, they also gave me a sense of security and reassurance that I was doing everything possible to stay healthy.

But follow-up care isn't just about physical health. It's also about addressing the emotional and psychological impact of cancer. Many survivors experience anxiety, depression, and other mental health issues in the aftermath of cancer, and it's important to have resources and support to address these concerns.

For me, follow-up care also included therapy and support groups where I could talk openly about my experience and connect with others who had been through a similar journey. These resources were invaluable in helping me to process my emotions and to navigate the challenges of life after cancer.

Ultimately, follow-up care is about taking ownership of your health and well-being. It's about being an active participant in your own care and staying vigilant about any changes or symptoms that may indicate a recurrence. And while it can be scary and overwhelming at times, it's also an opportunity to celebrate how far you've come and to look forward to a future filled with hope and possibility.

Embracing a New Sense of Purpose

Cancer is a life-changing experience that can completely alter the course of your life. For many survivors, the experience of cancer sparks a renewed sense of purpose and a desire to give back to others.

For me, this newfound sense of purpose came from the realization that I had been given a second chance at life. I felt a deep sense of gratitude for the support and care I had received throughout my cancer journey, and I wanted to pay it forward by helping others who were going through a similar experience.

One way I did this was by volunteering with cancer support organizations and advocacy groups. I found it incredibly fulfilling to use my experience to help others, whether it was by providing emotional support or by advocating for better cancer care and research.

Another way I found purpose was by pursuing new interests and hobbies that I had always been curious about but had never had the time or energy to explore. I started taking art classes, learning a new language, and even took up hiking. These activities gave me a sense of joy and fulfillment that helped me to move past the trauma of cancer and to embrace the present moment.

Ultimately, finding a new sense of purpose after cancer is about tapping into your own unique talents and passions, and using them to make a positive impact in the world. It's about recognizing the fragility of life and embracing the opportunities that come your way with a newfound sense of courage and resilience.

Conclusion

My cancer journey was one of the most challenging experiences of my life, but it was also one of the most transformative. Throughout the ups and downs of treatment, recovery, and life after cancer, I learned some valuable lessons that I will carry with me always.

The first lesson was the importance of self-care. Cancer treatment is grueling, both physically and emotionally, and it's important to prioritize your own well-being throughout the process. Whether it's getting enough rest, practicing mindfulness and relaxation techniques, or seeking out emotional support, taking care of yourself is essential to surviving and thriving through cancer.

The second lesson was the importance of community. Cancer can be an isolating experience, but it doesn't have to be. Building a support network of friends, family, and medical professionals can make all the difference in your journey. And connecting with others who have been through a similar experience can provide a sense of comfort and understanding that is hard to find elsewhere.

The third lesson was the importance of resilience. Cancer is a difficult journey, but it's also an opportunity to tap into your own strength and resilience. Learning to overcome challenges, to adapt to new circumstances, and to keep moving forward in the face of adversity can be incredibly empowering.

Finally, my cancer journey taught me the importance of gratitude. Gratitude for the support and care I received from loved ones and medical professionals. Gratitude for the simple pleasures of life, like a warm cup of tea or a walk in the park. And gratitude for the gift of life itself.

While cancer will always be a part of my story, it doesn't define me. Rather, it has taught me valuable lessons about what it means to live a meaningful, fulfilling life. And for that, I am forever grateful.

Words of Encouragement for Those Facing Cancer

To anyone who is facing cancer, I want to offer words of encouragement and hope. I know firsthand how difficult and overwhelming this journey can be, but I also know that it is possible to come out on the other side stronger and more resilient than ever before.

First and foremost, know that you are not alone. There are countless people who have been through a similar experience and are here to support you every step of the way. Reach out to friends, family, or support groups and let them be there for you. Don't be afraid to ask for help when you need it.

Secondly, remember to take care of yourself. This includes both your physical and emotional well-being. Eat well, get plenty of rest, and prioritize exercise and other self-care activities. Seek out professional help if you need it, whether that means counseling or medical treatment.

Finally, hold onto hope. Cancer can be a scary and uncertain journey, but there are also many success stories and reasons to remain optimistic. Focus on the present moment and take things one day at a time.

Celebrate even the smallest victories and milestones, and know that you have the strength and resilience to get through this.

Remember, cancer does not define you. It is only one part of your story, and you have the power to shape the rest of that story. Keep fighting, stay strong, and know that there is a community of people who are rooting for you every step of the way.

A Final Note of Gratitude

As I come to the end of this book, I want to take a moment to express my heartfelt gratitude. First and foremost, I am grateful for the opportunity to share my story with you. It is my hope that in reading about my journey, you have found comfort, inspiration, and hope.

I am also grateful for the countless individuals who have supported me along the way. To my family, friends, and healthcare team, thank you for your unwavering support and encouragement. Your love and kindness have sustained me through even the toughest moments.

Finally, I want to express my gratitude to the countless individuals who work tirelessly to advance cancer research and treatment. Your dedication and commitment are truly awe-inspiring, and I am grateful for all that you do to help those who are facing cancer.

In closing, I want to offer my best wishes to all those who are facing cancer or supporting someone who is. Remember that you are not alone, and that there is always hope. Keep fighting, stay strong, and know that there is a community of people who are here to support you every step of the way. Thank you for reading, and may you find peace and healing on your journey.

Appendix

Resources for Cancer Patients and Caregivers

If you or a loved one are facing cancer, there are many resources available to help you navigate this journey. Here are just a few:

1. American Cancer Society (ACS) - The ACS is a nationwide organization that provides support and resources for cancer patients and caregivers. They offer a helpline, support groups, and information about treatment options and financial assistance.

2. CancerCare - CancerCare is a national organization that provides free counseling, support groups, educational workshops, and financial assistance to cancer patients and their families.

3. National Cancer Institute (NCI) - The NCI is a government organization that conducts cancer research and provides information about cancer treatment and clinical trials. They also offer a helpline for patients and caregivers.

4. Livestrong Foundation - The Livestrong Foundation provides

resources and support for cancer patients and survivors, including counseling, support groups, and financial assistance.

5. Caregiver Action Network (CAN) - CAN is an organization that provides support and resources for caregivers of cancer patients. They offer educational resources, a helpline, and support groups.

6. Cancer Support Community (CSC) - The CSC provides support and resources for cancer patients and caregivers, including support groups, educational workshops, and counseling services.

7. Patient Advocate Foundation (PAF) - The PAF provides resources and support for patients with chronic or life-threatening illnesses, including cancer. They offer assistance with healthcare access, insurance issues, and financial assistance.

These are just a few of the many resources available to cancer patients and caregivers. Don't be afraid to reach out and ask for help - there are many people who are here to support you on this journey.

Glossary of Medical Terms

Here is a glossary of medical terms related to cancer:

1. Adenocarcinoma: a type of cancer that starts in cells that make up glands.

2. Biopsy: a procedure in which a small piece of tissue is removed for examination under a microscope.

3. Chemotherapy: treatment using drugs to kill cancer cells.

4. Clinical trial: a research study that tests new treatments for cancer.

5. Immunotherapy: treatment that stimulates the body's own immune system to fight cancer cells.

6. Metastasis: the spread of cancer cells from the original site of the cancer to other parts of the body.

7. Oncologist: a doctor who specializes in the diagnosis and treatment of cancer.

8. Palliative care: care that focuses on improving the quality of life for patients with serious illnesses, such as cancer.

9. Radiation therapy: treatment using high-energy radiation to kill cancer cells.

10. Remission: a period of time when the signs and symptoms of cancer disappear.

11. Tumor: an abnormal growth of cells that may be benign (not cancerous) or malignant (cancerous).

12. Staging: a system used to describe the extent and spread of cancer in the body.

13. Surgery: a procedure in which cancerous tissue is removed from the body.

14. Oncogene: a gene that, when mutated or overexpressed, can

contribute to the development of cancer.

15. Carcinogen: a substance or agent that can cause cancer.

16. Hormone therapy: treatment that blocks hormones or slows their production to stop or slow down the growth of cancer cells that rely on hormones to grow.

17. Neoplasm: a new and abnormal growth of tissue, which can be benign or malignant.

18. PET scan: a type of imaging test that uses a small amount of

radioactive material to produce detailed images of the inside of the body.

19. Prognosis: the expected outcome or chance of recovery from a disease, such as cancer.

20. Support group: a group of people who provide emotional and practical support for one another, often for those going through cancer treatment or those who have survived cancer.

21. Survivorship: the period of time after completing cancer treatment when a person is considered a cancer survivor.

22. Targeted therapy: treatment that targets specific genes, proteins, or other molecules that are involved in the growth and spread of cancer cells.

23. Ultrasound: a type of imaging test that uses high-frequency sound waves to produce images of the inside of the body.

24. Chemoprevention: the use of drugs, vitamins, or other substances to reduce the risk of cancer or the recurrence of cancer.

25. Genetic counseling: a process in which a person is given information about their risk of developing cancer based on their family history and genetic testing.

Remember, this glossary is not exhaustive, and there may be additional terms or treatments specific to your individual situation. Be sure to ask your healthcare provider for more information and clarification as needed.

Recommended Reading and Viewing

If you or a loved one is facing a colon cancer diagnosis, it can be helpful to read and watch informative materials to help you better understand the disease and treatment options. Here are a few recommended resources:

Books:

- "From Diagnosis to Remission: A Patient's Guide to Beating Colon Cancer by Dr. Gary A. Hudgins
- "Plant-Powered Cancer-Fighting Recipe: Delicious and Nutritions Meal to Combat Cancer by Theodore L. Acevedo
- "Radical Remission: Surviving Cancer Against All Odds" by Kelly Turner
- "When Breath Becomes Air" by Paul Kalanithi

Documentaries:

- "The C Word" (2016)
- "The Emperor of All Maladies" (2015)
- "A Time to Live" (2015)
- "Living Proof" (2017)
- "One Year Later" (2018)

Online Resources:

- The American Cancer Society (www.cancer.org)
- The National Cancer Institute (www.cancer.gov)
- The Colon Cancer Alliance (www.ccalliance.org)

- The Colorectal Cancer Coalition (www.coloncancercoalition.org)
- The Colon Cancer Foundation (www.coloncancerfoundation.org)

These resources can provide you with valuable information and support throughout your journey with colon cancer. Remember to always consult with your healthcare provider before making any decisions about your treatment.

9 798390 869468